DR SEBI

NATURAL

BLOOD

PRESSURE

CONTROL

Shobi Nolan

Contents

CHAPTER 1

INTRODUCTION

The measurement of blood pressure considers the amount of blood that passes through the blood vessels and the responding resistance to blood flow as the heart pumps blood. When the blood pressure increases too high to a level considered to be unhealthy, the condition is what is referred to as High Blood Pressure.

If you can remember high school physics where Boyle's law explains the relationship between volume and pressure - the lower the volume, the higher the pressure. The same principle holds between blood pressure and the size of arteries. Narrow arteries increase blood pressure because of increased resistance to blood flow.

However, if the blood pressure is high over the long term, it can lead to heart problems like heart disease, damaged blood vessels, and damaged organs like the brain, kidney, eyes, stroke, etc.

The symptoms of high blood pressure are not obvious,

especially at an early stage of the problem. Averagely, this can take many years to develop. Thus, almost half of American citizens are expected to be diagnosed with high blood pressure, since the guidelines were changed.

Detecting the issue early is vital to its management. And the best way to track blood pressure is through regular readings. Once detected early, it can be easily treated and managed. But if not treated immediately, the problem can cause severe health complications such as heart attack and stroke.

Symptoms of High Blood Pressure

High blood pressure is popularly known as the 'silent killer' because it doesn't have a noticeable symptom until the condition becomes severe. If not noticed, it can take years for the symptoms to be obvious, and by then the condition has become too severe and developed into other health problems.

Some of the conditions to watch out for are:

- Shortness of breath

- Dizziness

- Headache

- Chest pain

- Flushing

- Visual impairment

- Nosebleeds

- Blood in urine

Any of these symptoms of blood pressure needs urgent medical care. Though not all of them occur in everyone with high blood pressure, to wait for a symptom could be disastrous. So, it's important to visit the doctor on a regular basis for blood pressure reading.

Causes of High Blood Pressure

There are many factors that are responsible for hypertension. Each of these factors only causes a specific type of hypertension. There are two different cases of high blood pressure and each case has different factors causing it.

Types Of Hypertension And Their Causes:

Primary High Blood Pressure

This type of hypertension is known as essential hypertension. Most people you pass on the street every day have this kind of high blood pressure. It can develop over time without any symptoms.

There is no clear identifiable factor responsible for primary hypertension but research reports have made suggestions on the possible causes of this type of high blood pressure. Some of the factors include;

Physical Changes: Changes in your body may impact the blood flow rate in your system. Any change that makes the arteries to become narrow will affect the blood pressure. Not only that, but other changes that affect the chemical/fluid balance in the body can also alter blood pressure

Genes: Genetic abnormalities or mutations can be responsible for high blood pressure. Sometimes, they are inherited from parents.

Environment: Your surroundings and lifestyle matter a lot to your health. An unhealthy lifestyle is detrimental to your health and can lead to obesity, high cholesterol, stress, etc which can subsequently lead to high blood pressure.

Secondary High Blood Pressure

This type of hypertension occurs faster than primary hypertension and it is more severe. There are so many health factors that can cause this type of high blood pressure, some of which include:

- Congenital heart defect
- Thyroid problem
- Kidney problem
- Hard drugs
- Too much alcohol
- Obstructive sleep apnea
- Endocrine tumors
- Adrenal gland issue
- Some medications, etc.

CHAPTER 2

DIAGNOSIS

If you have not received any blood pressure report from your doctor for a long time, request for one. The blood pressure reading is one of the factors that are put into consideration in any medical test. Diagnosing high blood pressure as simply checking the reading of your blood pressure.

It is good to know that blood pressure is not constant. It varies throughout the day. Stress alone can alter blood pressure. So, the diagnosis of hypertension takes more than one test to conclude your true state of health. If the blood pressure is high on the first test, your doctor will request that you take another reading in a few days.

If it's still high on the second test, the doctor should arrange for another test. Some of these tests include;

- Cholesterol screening

- ECG

- Ultrasound of kidney or heart

- Urine teat

Once you detect high blood pressure early, start treating it immediately to avoid any risk of health damage.

Understanding High Blood Pressure Reading

Anyone can take a blood pressure reading. Once you understand the numbers, you can take blood pressure reading by yourself. It's still advisable to consult your doctor in anything related to your health.

There are two numbers, systolic and diastolic pressure, in

every blood pressure reading
instrument.

Systolic pressure: The first
number at the top of the screen
is the systolic pressure, which
measures the amount of pressure
on the arteries when your heart
pumps blood.

Diastolic pressure: The number
at the bottom of the scale is the
diastolic pressure that measures
the pressure on the arteries
between two consecutive
heartbeats.

Categories Of Blood Pressure

Blood pressure readings are grouped into 5 categories to help you determine how high or how low your blood pressure is. These categories are:

Healthy: Your blood pressure is healthy when the reading is below 120/80mmHg.

Elevated: Your blood pressure is considered elevated when the systolic number is within the range of 120 and 129mmHg while the diastolic number is below

80mmHg. Though it's considered high at this level, taking medication is not the best treatment approach. Changing your lifestyle will help to reduce the pressure.

Stage 1 Hypertension: Your blood pressure is considered to be in stage 1 hypertension when the systolic number is within the range of 130 to 139mmHg, or when the diastolic number ranges between 80 to 89mmHg.

Stage 2 hypertension: Your blood pressure is considered to be in stage 2 hypertension when the systolic reads 140mmHg or above, or when the diastolic reads 90mmHg or above.

Hypertensive Crisis: Your blood pressure is considered to be in Hypertension Crisis when the systolic reads above 180mmHg or when the diastolic reads above 120mmHg. At this level, emergency medical services are highly required. Some of the symptoms are headache, visual impairment, shortness of breath, chest pain, etc.

Note: *The ranges above are for adults. The blood pressure reading for children is different. Consult your child's doctor for directions. While taking blood pressure readings, it is important that you use a pressure cuff that fits well in order to get accurate results.*

CHAPTER 3

DR. SEBI DIET

Dr. Sebi's alkaline diet is a plant-based diet that helps to eliminate toxic wastes from the body and rejuvenate body cells.

The alkaline diet relies strictly on a list of plant foods and products approved by Dr. Sebi. Through his diet, Dr. Sebi did great wonders in people's lives; cured many diseases and revived complicated health conditions. In fact, it is one of the best plant-based diets. It was listed as one of the most popular diets in 2019.

If we can eat delicious meals and free our body from diseases, what again are we looking for? Dr. Sebi's diet can help you detox your body completely, including mucus removal, liver cleansing, diabetes reversal, cancer treatment, lupus and herpes cure, etc. Learn how to eat good foods, and you may not need medications to stay healthy.

You don't need medications to cleanse mucus from your body when you can easily get rid of it naturally by drinking and eating the right foods. By so doing, you can simply prevent and/or manage high blood pressure. The foods to take good care of your condition can be found in the nearest local grocery store.

Prepare your mind and stock your kitchen with the right foods from Dr. Sebi Approved List. Then follow the instructions in the book to help you lower your blood pressure.

But before we get started, let's look at Dr. Sebi and his diet.

Who is Dr. Sebi?

Alfredo Darlington Bowman is an African herbalist who developed an alkaline plant diet that is based on bio-mineral balance theory. Though he is not a certified medical doctor or a Ph.D. holder, he is widely known as Dr. Sebi.

His diet is named after his popular name, The Dr. Sebi Diet. His diet was developed for those that wish to naturally detox their body for total wellness and prevent diseases by eating approved healthy plant foods.

Dr. Sebi claimed that our body is protected from diseases

when it is in an alkaline state. According to him, acidic state of the body and mucus buildup in the body are the major causes of various diseases.

Though there is no scientific backup, Dr. Sebi claimed that his diet has the potential to cure lupus, sickle cell anemia, AIDS, and leukemia. He believes his diet could completely restore alkalinity in the body and detoxify the whole body.

Dr. Sebi Alkaline Diet

Dr. Sebi's diet is regarded as a vegan diet since it is a completely plant-based diet. No animal product is allowed in the diet.

Dr. Sebi claimed that this diet can make the body heal itself completely from diseases. Though there is no scientific proof for this, a lot of people who are on the diet have attested to the claim.

As a result, Dr. Sebi's diet is ranked one of the most popular diets in 2019.

The Dr. Sebi Diet Guide

Dr. Sebi's diet is solely based on plants and supplements approved by Dr. Sebi.

The diet guide can be found on his website. The simple rules to follow on Dr. Sebi diet are;

- Only foods and products listed in the nutritional guide are to be consumed.

- You must drink at least 1 gallon of water every day (that is about 3.8 liters).

- If you are on any medication, you have to take your Dr. Sebi supplements, at least, one hour before your medication.

- You don't take alcohol.

- You must not eat any animal products.

- Don't use the microwave to prepare your foods.

- Only consume naturally grown grains as listed in the guide. No wheat product is allowed.

- No seedless fruit and no canned food is permitted.

Moreover, you are expected to be using Dr. Sebi's supplements to support your diet.

CHAPTER 4

HIGH BLOOD PRESSURE AND PREGNANCY

Babies can be delivered safely without any health complications by women with high blood pressure if the condition is properly managed. Otherwise, both baby and mother could be exposed to health complications. The baby can be born prematurely or with very low birth weight. The mother also has a high risk of decreased kidney function.

A lot of women develop high blood pressure during pregnancy, which often reverses itself after delivery. But, if not properly managed, the condition may not reverse and can cause other health problems associated with hypertension.

Developing Pre-eclampsia

Some pregnant women with high blood pressure usually develop pre-eclampsia. This health issue may cause health problems in the body organs, high protein level, visual problem, defective liver function, lungs fluid, etc if it's not well managed. Moreover, it can progress to eclampsia that causes seizures.

Though there is no scientifically approved prevention method for pre-eclampsia, a healthy diet still remains the best prevention method for all diseases. But if any pregnant woman develops pre-eclampsia, the doctor has the responsibility of monitoring the condition closely.

CHAPTER 5

EFFECTS OF HIGH BLOOD PRESSURE

As a silent killer, hypertension can cause so many damages to the body without symptoms until the complications become severe. Some of the damages that high blood pressure can cause to the body include;

Damaged Heart: It is unhealthy to overwork the heart. Hypertension makes the muscles of the heart work so much by pumping more frequently with force due to the increased pressure on the blood vessels.

This can lead to heart enlargement which increases the risk of arrhythmia, heart failure, heart attack, and sudden cardiac death.

Damaged Arteries: Arteries are always strong and flexible which allows blood to flow freely without obstruction. But when the arteries become less elastic and tighter because of hypertension, It creates room for fats to deposit on it and this makes the arteries to be narrower for blood to flow freely.

This restriction to flood flow increases blood pressure and may cause stroke and heart attack.

Damaged Brain: The brain cannot function properly without oxygen-rich blood. High blood pressure can limit the flow of oxygen-rich blood to the brain which causes brain cells to die - stroke.

Moreover, it can lead to memory loss, inability to speak, or reason properly.

CHAPTER 6

HOW TO LOWER HIGH BLOOD PRESSURE

Exercise More

A study carried out in 2013 has shown that increased activity can help to lower blood pressure. In the study, the systolic and diastolic pressure of old people that took part in aerobic training reduced by an average of 3.9 and 4.5 percent, respectively. Some medications cannot perform more than this.

Regular exercise helps the heart to pump blood at a normal rate with less effort. This helps to lower blood pressure.

According to the American Heart Association (AHA) and the American College of Cardiology (ACC), regular 40 minutes sessions of moderate or vigorous-intensity exercise of about 4 times a week are good for a healthy heart. This report was also recommended by the American College of Sports Medicine (ACSM).

Some simple activities one can do to cover this activity rate include,

- Biking

- Gardening

- Swimming

- Jumping

- Walking

- Running, etc.

Just find something that can keep your body busy and active for a period of time. Climbing stairs is even okay. In another study on Tai Chi and blood pressure, the systolic and diastolic pressure of people that participate reduced by an average of 15.6mmHg and 10.7mmHg, respectively.

Another review in 2014 shows that 10,000 footsteps a day can help to lower high blood pressure.

Weight Loss

Research has shown that 5 - 10lb of weight loss can help to lower blood pressure. Moreover, it will also help to reduce the risk of developing other health problems.

Lower Your Sugar Intake

Cutting refined carbohydrates and sugar from your daily diet can help in weight loss and reduction of blood pressure.

Different studies have shown that a low-carb diet is highly effective in lowering blood pressure more than a low-fat diet.

Reduce Sodium and Increase Potassium In Your Diet

Potassium helps to ease tension in the blood vessels. It also helps to lower the effects of salt in the body. Therefore, lowering sodium and increasing potassium intake can help to lower blood pressure.

There are so many Dr. Sebi approved foods that are rich in potassium such as avocados, bananas, oranges, greens, etc.

Don't Eat Processed Foods

Salt and some chemicals used to make and preserve processed food can alter the blood pressure level.

Just as Dr. Sebi directed, cut it off completely from your diet.

Stop Smoking

Smoking is not good for anyone. Smoking can affect the entire body badly and increases health risks. It can damage the walls of the blood vessels and causes the arteries to become narrow. This damage in turn causes the blood pressure to increase.

However, following Dr. Sebi diet means that you will quit smoking. To read further on smoking and learn how to quit smoking easily using Dr. Sebi guide, get a copy of ***Dr Sebi Easy Way To Stop Smoking***

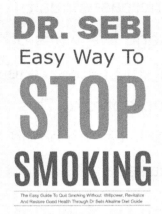

DR. SEBI
Easy Way To
STOP
SMOKING

The Easy Guide To Quit Smoking Without Willpower, Revitalize
And Restore Good Health Through Dr Sebi Alkaline Diet Guide

Shobi Nolan

Link to kindle edition:
https://www.amazon.com/dp/B0
8J9QNZBR

Link to print edition:
https://www.amazon.com/SEBI-
EASY-WAY-STOP-
SMOKING/dp/B08JF5CZBZ

Avoid Stress

Nowadays, it seems impossible to live each day without stress. There are so many distractions here and there. But no matter how it turns out, we must find a way to go about it because excess stress is detrimental to our health. There are some activities we can do to relieve the nerves from stress. These activities include:

- Listening to music

- Watching comedy shows

- Reading books

- Doing breathing exercises

- Meditation, etc.

Research has shown that these activities help to reduce blood pressure.

Take More Herbs

Herbs have been used since ancient times to treat different ailments. Herbs are so beneficial in so many ways. Some herbs such as sesame and ginger are used to reverse high blood pressure in some cultures.

Sleep Well

A study on sleep and heart health revealed that regular sleep below 7 hours or above 9 hours a night may cause hypertension. 5 hours of sleep or less is linked to a high risk of hypertension.

Sleep helps to lower blood pressure. So, don't deprive yourself of that.

Fresh Garlic (optional)

Though garlic is not one of the approved foods by Dr. Sebi, it is highly effective in lowering high blood pressure as studies have shown.

Eat More Protein And High-Fiber Content Foods

Research reports have shown that regular consumption of 100g of protein can reduce the risk of hypertension by 40 percent while regular fiber intake lowers the risk by 60 percent.

Take Dr. Sebi Herbal Teas

Dr. Sebi's herbal teas have helped thousands of people to restore good health. Products like Dr. Sebi's Blood Pressure Balance Herbal Tea and Dr. Sebi's Nerve / Stress Relief Herbal Tea can help to lower cholesterol, induce sleep, and regulate blood pressure.

Say No To Alcohol

Alcohol is known as one of the drinks that raise blood pressure. About 10 grams of alcohol can increase your blood pressure by 1mmHg. Therefore, there is no need to take alcohol since all we want is a reduction in blood pressure. Besides, alcohol is highly restricted in Dr. Sebi's diet. Also, avoid caffeine. Learn Dr. Sebi's complete guide on how to quit drinking alcohol easily in **Dr**

Sebi Easy Guide To Stop Drinking Alcohol

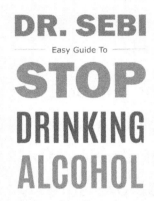

Link to kindle edition:

https://www.amazon.com/dp/B0 8KH2L5RZ

Take Medications As Prescribed By Your Doctor

If you must take any medication ensure it's from your doctor's prescription. Never take a drug unless it's recommended by your doctor, or you are a health practitioner.

Some Medications Used To Lower High Blood Pressure.

Alpha-2 Agonists: These medicines alter the nerve impulse that tightens the blood vessels. They help to relax the blood vessels and lower blood pressure.

Angiotensin Converting Enzyme (ACE) Inhibitors:

Angiotensin tightens and narrows the walls of the blood vessels and arteries. ACE inhibitors inhibit the enzymes from producing the chemical.

Beta-blockers: beta-blockers lower the production of hormones that are responsible for increased blood pressure. They also slow down the heart beat and lower the amount of blood that flows through the arteries. This helps to lower blood pressure.

Calcium Channel Blockers: These medicines limit the amount of calcium that goes to the cardiac muscles of the heart. Limited supply of calcium makes the heartbeat to be less forceful and thus, lowers blood pressure.

ARBs: Unlike the ACE inhibitors that prevent production of angiotensin, Angiotensin II Receptor Blockers prevents the enzyme from binding with its receptor.

Diuretics: Also known as water pills, diuretics help the kidneys to remove any excess sodium that accumulates in the body. This process removes any extra fluid in the bloodstream through urine, and thus lowers blood pressure.

Note: *Before you use any of the medications listed above, make sure you work with your doctor to know the one that will work best for you.*

If you have the Dr. Sebi product(s), make sure you take them at least one hour before you take any pharmaceuticals.

CHAPTER 7

DR SEBI VEGETABLES THAT LOWER BLOOD PRESSURE

Foods with high water content and/or fiber can help the body stay hydrated, and hence prevent and cleanse excess mucus in the body. The Dr. Sebi vegetables are awesome foods with high amount of water and fiber content.

Taking these veggies will not only help you cleanse mucus, they will help your body to detox and heal naturally.

Below are some of the veggies and ways you can add them to your diet for a super healthy living.

Tomato (The Plum And Cherry)

Scientific Name: *Solanum lycopersicum*

Overview

Tomato is a popular plant grown all over the world in a temperate climate. It's widely used in different cuisines. Though it's native to western South America, China, India, the United States, and Turkey are currently the highest producers of tomatoes.

Tomato is used in many ways because of its umami flavor. It can be taken raw or cooked.

Major Compounds

Beta-carotene, lutein zeaxanthin, thiamine, niacin, vitamin B-6, vitamin C, vitamin E, vitamin K, magnesium, manganese, phosphorus, potassium

Health benefits

Heart health: Tomatoes contain high amounts of potassium and fiber. These components are important for keeping the heart healthy. Fiber helps the body to reduce cholesterol level in the blood. High consumption of potassium helps to lower the blood pressure which is good for the heart.

Healthy bone: Phosphorus, magnesium, and vitamin C play crucial roles in the development of string and healthy bones. Tomatoes contain high amounts of phosphorus and moderate amounts of magnesium and vitamin C.

Eye health: The lutein and beta-carotene found in tomatoes are needed by our eyes to protect the retina and keep the eye free from macular degeneration.

Prevents cancer: tomatoes contain several vitamins and antioxidants such as lycopene, beta-carotene, vitamin C, etc. These components have properties that enables them to fight cancer cells and free radicals that can cause damage to the body cells.

How To Use

Tomatoes are used in many ways. It can be eaten raw or cooks. It can be used to make side dishes. Awesome for fruit and vegetable salads. Tomorrow is the major ingredient for stew. Many use it to cook soup, make sandwiches, or add it to wraps.

There are so many ways to use it. It can be used for smoothies and juice.

Nutrition fact

Per 100g

- Calories: 18 kcal

- Carbs: 3.9g

- Sugars: 2.6g

- Fiber: 1.2g

- Fat: 0.2g

- Protein: 0.9g

Side Effects

Excessive intake of tomatoes can lead to some unhealthy conditions. Some of these side effects include diarrhea, acid reflux, headache, kidney stones, lycopenodermia, joint pain, severe throat/mouth irritation, vomiting, mild spasms, dizziness, etc.

NOTE

Squash

Scientific Name: *Cucurbita spp.*

Overview

Squash is a widely used food crop that originated from Mexico. Now popular in the South, North America, and Asia. India and China have been the highest producers of squash so far.

There are different types of squashes with several color variations. Squash has fed many mouths and is still feeding a lot at the moment. It is cooked and used in different dishes.

Major Compounds

Beta-carotene, lutein, zeaxanthin, thiamine, riboflavin, niacin, pantothenic acid, vitamin B6, folate, vitamin C, vitamin K, iron, magnesium, manganese, phosphorus, potassium, zinc, oleic, palmitic, and linoleic fatty acids.

Health benefits

Heart health: Fiber and potassium are important substances that help to take care of the heart. High fiber content foods help to reduce the cholesterol level in our blood.

Enough intake of potassium helps the body to lower blood pressure. Squash contains a high amount of potassium which is vital to the heart.

Cancer: squash contains important antioxidants that may help the body to prevent cancer. Some of these antioxidants reduce the growth rate of cancer cells and help to protect the body cells against free radicals.

Healthy Eye: Squash contains beta-carotene and lutein, which are important compounds for healthy eyes. They help to protect the retina and keep the eyes free from macular degeneration.

How To Use

Simply wash and peel off the skin. Then use as you desire. You can cook your squash, or roast it. Smashed and used as an ingredient for other dishes like soup.

Some squash have tough cover. To peel them off you need to put them in your oven for about 2 minutes, with the skin pierced with a fork. Or bake/cook with the skin on. Then it will be easier to remove the skin.

Nutrition fact

Per 100g

- Calories: 16 kcal

- Carbs: 3.4g

- Sugars: 2.2g

- Fiber: 1.1g

- Fat: 0.2g

- Protein: 1.2g

Side Effects

Some of the side effects associated with the use of squash

include allergic reactions such as dermatitis, itching, difficulty in breathing, nasal congestion, swelling of face and lips, etc.

NOTE

Onion

Scientific Name: *Allium cepa*

Overview

Onion is one of the most popular food ingredients used worldwide. Though its origin has many claims, the only fact is that onion originated from Asia.

It is widely cultivated all over the world. It can be eaten raw or cooked. Onion can be pungent to the eye when exposed. Three types of onions are predominant; the yellow onion, red onion, and white onion. All

are flavorful and super healthy
for use.

Major Compounds
Polyphenols, thiamine, riboflavin,
niacin, pantothenic acid, vitamin
B-6, folate, vitamin C, calcium,
iron, magnesium, manganese,
phosphorus, potassium, zinc

Health benefits
Cancer: the antioxidants in
onions can help the body to fight
against cancer by protecting the
body cells against oxidative
damage. They can reduce the

growth of cancer cells, and thus, helps to reduce the risk of cancer.

Heart health: fiber in our foods helps to lower the level of cholesterol in our body. Moreover, the high amount of potassium in onions plays a vital role in the reduction of blood pressure. These properties of onions plus more ensure a healthy heart.

Osteoporosis: Calcium, potassium, and vitamin C are important to the bone. These compounds provided in good amounts by onion can help the body to develop strong and healthy bones.

Anti-inflammatory: Destroying radical cells that are toxic to the body is one of the means our body uses to prevent inflammation. The antioxidants from onions help the body to fight against these radicals.

How To Use

Onion is used to prepare most dishes.

First peel off the outer layer and wash. Dice or slice to your taste and add to your food; salads, wraps, sandwiches, soup, stew, etc. It can be taken raw or cooked. Anyway, it is super healthy for consumption.

Nutrition fact

Per 100g

- Calories: 40
- Fat: 0.1g
- Carbs: 9g
- Fiber: 1.7g
- Sugar: 4.2g
- Protein: 1.1g

Side Effects

Some of the side effects associated with the use of onions include blurred vision, dermatitis, bronchial asthma, itching, sweating, and anaphylaxis

NOTE

Okra

Scientific Name: *Abelmoschus esculentus*

Overview

Okra is a widely used vegetable all over the world. Some regions call it Okro or ladies' finger. This healthy plant that originated from West Africa has a mucilaginous property. This makes most foods cooked with okra to be slimy, unless it's deslimed. One of the things mostly used to deslime okra is tomato.

This healthy vegetable is widely cultivated for food because of its nutritional values. It is used in many ways such as in making salads, soups, stews, etc.

Major Compounds

Protein, carbohydrates, fiber, vitamin K, vitamin C, thiamin, folate, magnesium, riboflavin, niacin, potassium, calcium, iron, phosphorus, zinc, flavonoids, and isoquercetin

Health benefits

Prevention of Cancer: okra contains lectin and folate. Researches suggest that these compounds strongly inhibit the growth of cancer cells. Thus, taking enough okra can help one to prevent the risk of cancer.

Pregnancy: The folate gotten from okra helps to keep a healthy pregnancy. Lack of folate in the body may possibly lead to miscarriage.

Prevents diabetes: Test done on animals (rat) shows that okra can reduce the fat and blood sugar level in the body.

Heart health: Okra provides the body with useful fibers which can help to keep the heart-healthy. American Heart Association (AHA) suggests that food with high fiber content helps the body to reduce cholesterol level.

Osteoporosis: okra provides a high amount of calcium and vitamin K to the body. Calcium and vitamin K are very vital for the development of strong and healthy bones.

How To Use

Okra can be used in many ways. It can be taken raw, roasted, pickled, fried, boiled, or sauteed. You can add it to your soup, salads, or other foods.

To remove the sliminess of okra in your food, try and cook it over high heat and avoid cooking in a crowded pot. You can also pickle it or cook with acidic food like tomato.

Nutrition fact

Per 100g

- Calories: 33

- Fat: 0.2g

- Carbs: 7g

- Fiber: 3.2g

- Sugar: 1.5g

- Protein: 1.9g

Side Effects

Some side effects associated with the use of okra include cramping, diarrhea, gas, and bloating.

NOTE

Nopals

Scientific Name: *Opuntia spp.*

Overview

Native to Mexico, nopales is a food ingredient with important health benefits. There are about 114 species of nopales in Mexico. This highly medicinal food is not popular like other herbs such as lettuces, kale, etc, but it is common among the residents of southwest America.

It's popularly known in English as "prickly pear".

Major Compounds

Manganese, vitamin C, magnesium, calcium, antioxidants, sodium, potassium

Health benefits

Antiviral: research suggests that nopales gas antiviral properties that can be used against herpes and HIV.

Antioxidant: Nopales have a high content of antioxidants which help to protect the body cells against radical damage and reduce oxidative stress.

Blood Sugar Level: research has it that nopales have important properties that can help to regulate blood sugar levels.

Cholesterol: earlier studies suggest that nopales can lower cholesterol levels, especially LDL cholesterol.

Enlarged Prostate: Nopales may help to reduce enlarged prostate, which is a serious health condition for men. It may as well help to treat prostate cancer.

How To Use

Nopales can be eaten raw or cooked. It can be used to make juice, jams, smoothies, tea, etc.

It can be prepared with other Dr. Sebi approved foods as side dishes, salads, etc.

Nutrition fact
Per 100g

- Calories: 16

- Total Fat: 0.1g

- Fiber: 2g

- Sugar: 1.1g

- Protein: 1.4g

Side Effects

Some of the side effects associated with nopales include bloating, headache, diarrhea, nausea

NOTE

Mushrooms

Scientific Name: *Agaricus bisporus*

Overview

With over 14,000 types, mushrooms are widely cultivated all over the world for commercial and medicinal use. China, Italy, and the United States are known to be among the highest producers of mushrooms.

The most consumed mushroom until this century remains the white mushrooms. There are many health benefits associated with mushrooms and that is one of the major reasons why it gained its popularity.

However, not all mushrooms are edible as some can be highly toxic to the body. There are over 2,000 edible mushrooms. Among the edible ones shiitake is not approved for the Dr Sebi diet. So, it's pertinent that one should avoid shitake and any other mushroom that is not edible.

Major Compounds
Protein, pantothenic acid, riboflavin, niacin, copper, calcium, selenium, potassium, fiber,

vitamin D, ergothioneine,
glutathione

Health benefits

Cancer Prevention: The
antioxidants in mushrooms can
help to prevent cancer cells from
reproducing. Thus, mushrooms
help the body to lower the risk of
cancer.

Neurodegenerative Disease

(Alzheimer's): Ergothioneine
and glutathione which are
majorly produced by mushrooms
are claimed to be potentially
useful for the treatment of

Alzheimer's and Parkinson's diseases

Heart Health: Mushrooms are one of the major producers of potassium. High intake of potassium helps to reduce blood pressure.

Diabetes: The fiber content of mushrooms can help to fight against diabetes. Fiber is known to be useful in managing type 2 diabetes.

How To Use

First trim the end of the stalk, clean, and wash before use. It can be sliced, diced, or used the whole. Though it can be taken raw, cooked mushrooms are most preferred.

Mushrooms can be used to make salads, side dishes, pizza, scrambles, quiche, omelette, sandwiches, wraps, etc.

Nutrition fact

Per 100g

- Calories: 22

- Fat: 0.3g

- Total Carbs: 3.3g

- Fiber: 1g

- Sugar: 2g

- Protein: 3.1g

Side Effects

Dryness of the mouth or throat, rashes, diarrhea, itchiness, stomach upset, cramps, headache, nausea, vomiting, and diarrhea

NOTE

Dandelion

Scientific Name: *Taraxacum officinale*

Overview

Dandelion is a herbaceous plant grown all over the world for food and medicinal purposes. It's claimed to have a myriad of medicinal properties that can be used in the prevention and potential cure for physical ailments.

Native to North America and Eurasia, dandelion is widely consumed as a nutritious food. All parts of the plant are edible, including the flower, leaves, roots, and stems.

The flowers are known to contain high amounts of phytochemicals, with the leaves rich in lutein, while the root has a lot of probiotic fibers.

Major Compounds

Vitamin A, folate, vitamin K, vitamin C, calcium, potassium, iron, manganese, polyphenols, inulin, lutein, beta-carotene

Health benefits

Good Source of Antioxidants:

dandelion provides the body with

a good amount of antioxidants such as beta-carotene and polyphenols which help to protect the body cells against radical damages.

Regulation of Cholesterol Levels: researches done on animals suggests that dandelion is very effective in reducing cholesterol levels. It also lowers the amount of fat in the liver, which means that dandelion can be used for the treatment of fatty liver disease.

Blood Sugar Regulation: the antihyperglycemic, anti-inflammatory and antioxidative properties found in dandelion can be useful for the treatment of type 2 diabetes.

Anti-inflammatory: chemical extracts from dandelion are claimed to be potent in the reduction of body inflammation.

Blood Pressure Regulation: potassium is known to be an effective supplement for lowering blood pressure.

Weight Loss: the chlorogenic acid found in dandelion can be effective in reducing weight and lipid accumulation.

Prevention of Cancer: Research suggests that dandelion can be highly effective in the prevention of cancer as it has the potential to inhibit the growth of cancer cells.

Immune System Boost: The antibacterial and antiviral properties of dandelion can be useful for the immune system. Research suggests that dandelion can inhibit the growth of hepatitis B.

How To Use

Dandelion can be used in many ways. Depending on how you want it, it's mostly preferred when blanched to remove some bitterness. It can be taken raw (both fresh and dried), added to smoothies, teas, and juice, or used to make salads. It can be added to soup. The root can be roasted and used as coffee.

Nutrition fact

Per 100g

- Calories: 45

- Total Fat: 0.7g

- Total Carbs: 9.2g

- Fiber: 3.5g

- Sugar: 0.7g

- Protein: 2.7g

Side Effects

There is no enough record on the side effect on the use of dandelions. But dandelion can cause allergic reactions, diarrhea, or heartburn.

NOTE

Lettuce

Scientific Name: *Lactuca sativa*

Overview

Lettuce which originated from Egypt and mostly produced in China is widely known for its wonderful health benefits. Some people call it the perfect weight-loss food.

It can be used in diverse ways for various purposes, especially for medicinal purposes. In many regions, it is used for the treatment of typhoid, body pain, smallpox, rheumatism, coughs, and nervousness - even insanity, though there is no scientific backup for this claim.

There are different types of lettuce which include leaf lettuce, romaine lettuce, iceberg, summercrip, butterhead, red leaf, oilseed, and celtuce.

Note: Iceberg is not approved by Dr. Sebi.

Major Compounds

Vitamin K, vitamin A (beta-carotene, lutein, zeaxanthin), folate, iron, thiamine, riboflavin, pantothenic acid, vitamin c, vitamin e, calcium, magnesium, manganese, phosphorus, potassium, sodium, zinc

Health benefits
Prevents Dehydration: lettuce, especially red lettuce is made up of 96% water. This can help to keep the body hydrated.

Antioxidant: lettuce contains a lot of antioxidants such as beta-carotene which helps to protect the body cells against radical damage. Antioxidants play vital roles in the wholesome wellness of our bodies.

Heart Health: the presence of potassium in lettuce may help to lower the level of blood pressure.

Eye Health: The beta-carotene and other antioxidants got from lettuce help to protect the eye from macular degeneration.

Prevents Diabetes: Lettuce has a low glycemic index and zero glycemic loads which are good for those trying to lower their blood sugar, especially for managing type 2 diabetes.

How To Use

First wash the lettuce, pound on a chopping board to make it soft. Separate the leaves and dry.
Then tear into smaller parts and dress.

Lettuce can be used to make smoothies, salads, and sandwiches. It can also be added to soups and wraps.

Nutrition fact

Per 100g

- Calories: 15

- Fat: 0.2g

- Carbs: 2.9g

- Fiber: 1.3g

- Sugar: 0.8g

- Protein: 1.4g

Side Effects

Some of the potential side effects associated with lettuce consumption include sweating, itching, fast heartbeat, nausea, vomiting, pupil dilation, diarrhea, dizziness, ringing in the ears, vision rashes, vision changes, sedation, and breathing difficulty.

NOTE

Kale

Scientific Name: _Brassica oleracea_

Overview

Kale is one of the most popular veggies in the world. It is highly nutritious and heavily used for its medicinal properties.

It's claimed to originate from Asia Minor and Eastern Mediterranean where it was cultivated for food. Kale is best cultivated in the winter times for maximum yield.

Major Compounds

Protein, fiber, vitamins A, C, and K, folate, alpha-linolenic acid, lutein and zeaxanthin, phosphorus, potassium, calcium, zinc, carotenoids, phenols

Health benefits

Diabetes: The fiber content of kale can play an important role in the prevention and treatment of diabetes since fiber helps to regulate blood sugar level.

Antioxidants: kale contains a high amount of antioxidants which help to protect the body cells against oxidative damage.

Heart health: high intake of potassium and reduction in the consumption of sodium helps to lower the risk of high blood pressure. Moreover, fiber in our diet helps to lower cholesterol level. These properties help to take care of the heart.

Prevention Cancer: The presence of antioxidants in our body helps to protect our cells and hinder the development of cancer cells.

Healthy Eye: the lutein and zeaxanthin gotten from kale help to protect our eyes against macular degeneration. Vitamins, zinc, and beta-carotene help to protect the retina and keep the eyes healthy.

Healthy Bone: Calcium and vitamin K are very important for the development of healthy bones. Even, phosphorus and vitamin D also support the health of our bones.

Healthy skin and Hair: the human skin needs beta-carotene and vitamin A for development and maintenance of body tissues. Also, the vitamin C provided by kale helps to build and support the protein, collagen, responsible for skin and hair growth

How To Use

You can use kale in many ways. Kale can be eaten raw, steamed, or sauteed. Gently scrunch the kale leaf to make it soft. Then add it to your salads, sandwiches, and smoothies, wraps. Blend with other veggies and fruits to make smoothies and juice. Saute with onion for a side dish. You can spice it up and bake for 15-30 minutes to make your kale chips.

Nutrition fact

Per 100g

- Calories: 49

- Fat: 0.9g

- Total Carbs: 9g

- Protein: 4.3g

Side Effects

If you are battling with hypothyroidism, kale is not the best vegetable for you. Consult your physician for your diets. Excessive intake of kale can inhibit the production of thyroid hormone.

NOTE

Chayote

Scientific Name: *Sechium edule*

Overview

Chayote originated from Mexico and many parts of Latin America. Now it's grown all over the world. It's also known as choko or mirliton. It is mainly used when cooked.

Almost all part of this pear-shaped plant is edible, including the root, leaves, stem, and seeds. It contains loads of nutrients that can help transform and keep the body healthy.

Major Compounds

Potassium, vitamin C, magnesium, folate, manganese, vitamin K, vitamin B-6, zinc, quercetin, myricetin, morin, kaem pferol

Health benefits

Promotes Heart Health:

according to researchers, some chayote compounds help to reduce blood pressure and improve blood flow.

Also, Myricetin which is provided by the body helps to reduce the level of cholesterol in the body.

Moreover, taking fiber-rich foods helps to lower the risk of heart disease - chayote is one of the fiber-rich foods.

Blood Sugar Control: the fiber content of chayote helps to promote insulin sensitivity and regulation of blood sugar.

Support Healthy Pregnancy: The folate provided by chayote helps to lower the risk of miscarriage during pregnancy.

Anticancer: the myricetin in chayote has a strong anticancer property which helps to fight against cancer.

Anti-Aging: Chayote is loaded with a high amount of antioxidants which help to protect the body cells against oxidative damage. Also, since vitamin C is verily vital in the production of collagen, the high amount of vitamin C in chayote ensures the skin stays firm and youthful.

Prevents Liver Disease:
Excessive deposits of fats in the

liver leads to fatty liver disease. Test tube and animal studies suggest that chayote extract can help to protect the liver by preventing the accumulation of fats in the liver.

Support Digestion: The fiber and flavonoids from chayote keep the digestive tract healthy as they keep the digestive enzymes in the gut healthy and remove wastes from the digestive tract, respectively.

How To Use

Chayote is mainly used when cooked, roasted, steamed, or fried. You can also eat it raw by adding it to your salads and smoothies.

You can add it to stews, soups, casserole dishes.

Nutrition fact

Per 100g

- Calories: 19

- Fat: 0.1g

- Cholesterol: 0mg

- Sodium: 2mg

- Potassium: 125mg

- Carbs: 4.5g

- Fiber: 1.7g

- Sugar: 1.7 g

- Protein: 0.8 g

Side Effects

Allergic reactions

NOTE

Arugula

Scientific Name: *Eruca vesicaria*

Overview

Native to the Mediterraneans, arugula is a leafy green vegetable with fresh, bitter, tart, and peppery-mustard flavor. It is popularly known is some regions as garden rocket, roquette, rucola, or colewort. It is widely used as healthy ingredient for salads.

It is super nutrition and may help the body to prevent the risk of cancer, eye damage, or osteoporosis and arthritis.

Major Compounds

Potassium, calcium, phosphorus, vitamin k, vitamin b-6, vitamin c, magnesium, sodium, thiamine, riboflavin, dietary fiber, fat, protein, vitamin a, beta-carotene, lutein zeaxanthin, niacin, vitamin e, iron,

Health Benefits

Healthy Bone: Calcium, vitamin K, magnesium, and phosphorus supplied by arugula are the major minerals for the development of strong and healthy bone. These minerals helps the body to prevent any risk of osteoporosis and arthritis.

129

Heart Health: Arugula contains wonderful minerals to take care of the body naturally. Arugula contains high amount of potassium, vitamins and antioxidants, with moderate amount of fiber which help to protect the heart. The fiber helps the body to lower and regulate the level of cholesterol in the blood, while the potassium reduces blood pressure.

Cancer: The vitamins and antioxidants from arugula help the body to prevent the formation of cancer cells. They also protect the body cells against radical damage. This also aids anti-inflammation.

Eye Health: The high content of vitamin A, lutein and b-carotene in arugula protect and help the eyes to fight against macular degeneration.

How To Use

First rinse with cold water and dry. In addition to the leaves and seeds, it is good to know that the young seed pods, and flowers of arugula are also edible. They can be used to make salads. It can be added to soups, or used to make sauce. Some people also use it for their pizza.

Side Effects

Some possible side effects with excessive consumption of arugula include abdominal cramping, flatulence, and discomfort.

NOTE

Turnip Greens

Scientific Name: *Brassica rapa var. rapa*

Overview

Turnip greens are root vegetables widely cultivated worldwide as food crop. It thrives better in the temperate climates. Turnip green is known as one of the best sources of vitamins and regarded as one of the healthiest vegetables in the world.

During winter and late autumn, turnip is the most common side dish in southeastern region of United

States. It's fully packed with antioxidants, potassium, calcium, and fiber.

Major Compounds

potassium, phosphorus, magnesium, vitamin K, folate, vitamin C, zinc, iron, sodium, Lutein, beta-Carotene,

Health Benefits

Heart Health: Turnip contains wonderful substances to take care of the body naturally. Turnip contains high amount of potassium, fiber, vitamins and antioxidants which help to protect the heart. The fiber helps the body to lower and regulate the level of cholesterol in the blood, while the potassium is a good mineral used by the body to reduce blood pressure.

Hair and Skin Care: Vitamin C in one of the major vitamins supplied by turnip to the body. Vitamin C helps the body to build and maintain collagen. Vitamin A is vital for all body tissues including those for skin and hair. While iron helps to stop hair loss.

Healthy Bone: Calcium, vitamin K, vitamin D, magnesium, and phosphorus supplied by turnip are the major minerals for the development of strong and healthy bone. These minerals helps the body to prevent any risk of osteoporosis.

Pregnancy Care: The vitamins and minerals produced by turnip are vital to keep a healthy pregnancy. Folate in the body protects pregnant women from the risk of miscarriage.

Cancer: The vitamins and antioxidants from turnip helps the to prevent the development of cancer cells. They also protect the body cells against free radical which could cause serious damage to body cells. This also aids anti-inflammation.

Eye Health: The high content of lutein and b-carotene protects and helps fight against macular degeneration.

Diabetes: Fiber is known to help in managing type 2 diabetes as it helps to regulate blood sugar.

How To Use

First rinse with cold water, and slice as desired. Turnip can be eaten raw or cooked. You can add turnip to your salad or smoothie. It can be sauteed or boiled, and added to soups, casserole, or other dishes. Side dish for rice and beans,

Side Effects

Though turnip is a wonderful source of healthy minerals, too much consumption of it may not be healthy for the body since it contains high amount of these minerals already.

Some of the possible side effects that could be associated with the consumption of turnip include runny nose, cough, watery eyes, lip swelling and redness, sore eyes, sinus, breathing problems, etc.

NOTE

Watercress

Scientific Name: _Nasturtium officinale_

Overview

Watercress is a rapid growing flowering plant that is widely used in Europe and Asia. It is native to these two continents, but has found its wide use in other regions like the Americas. It is known to be one of the oldest vegetables on earth.

It is an aquatic plant and thus, perfect for hydroponic cultivation. It is used in different delicacies and it is highly nutritious. It can be eaten raw or cooked.

Major Compounds

potassium, calcium, vitamin K, phosphorus, folate, magnesium, vitamin C, vitamin A, beta-Carotene, lutein zeaxanthin, vitamin E, riboflavin, vitamin B-6, manganese, thiamine, pantothenic acid, iron, sodium

Health Benefits

Heart Health: Watercress contains high amount of potassium, vitamins and antioxidants which may help to keep a healthy heart. High amount of potassium helps the body to reduce blood pressure.

Skin Care: Vitamin C helps the body to build and maintain collagen while vitamin A is vital for tissue development including those for skin.

Healthy Bone: Calcium, vitamin K, vitamin C, and phosphorus from watercress are essential minerals in the formation of strong and healthy bone. These minerals keeps the bones free from osteoporosis and arthritis.

Cancer: The vitamins and antioxidants from turnip helps to prevent the build up of cancer cells. They also protect the body cells against oxidative damage to body cells.

Eye Health: The amount of lutein and b-carotene in watercress is very high and they can help to protect the eye from macular degeneration.

Other Possible Health Benefits

Some people use watercress as a short-term solution for inflammation of the lungs, baldness, and sexual arousal.

How To Use

Mostly used to make salads, watercress can be used in other foods like soup, omelet, scrambled egg, pasta sauce. It can be added to sandwiches, wraps, smoothies, and juice.

Side Effects

There is no enough record on the possible side effects of watercress. It is advisable to use moderate amount of watercress, and then watch out for any possible side effects.

NOTE

Purslane

Scientific Name: *Portulaca oleracea*

Overview

Purslane is a leafy green vegetable with sour and salty taste. Wide known as weed because of its ability to survive in harsh conditions, unlike other green veggies. It is more common as edible vegetable in the Middle East, Europe, and Asia. Even the Mexicans are used to it.

It can be eaten raw as salad or used in several delicacies. Its

mucilaginous property makes it
perfect for soups and stews.

Major Compounds

potassium, calcium, magnesium,
phosphorus, folate, vitamin B-6,
vitamin E, vitamin C, vitamin A,
iron, manganese, thiamine, niacin,
riboflavin, zinc

Health Benefits

Anti-inflammatory: The
vitamins gotten from purslane
have anti-inflammatory and
antioxidant properties. These
properties help to protect body
cells against free radicals and

thus, keep the body free from inflammation. It may also be essential for cancer prevention.

Heart Health: Purslane is one of the best sources of potassium among leafy greens. Thus, may be essential for the heart, since potassium helps to reduce blood pressure.

Skin Care: Vitamin C and E the major vitamins supplied by purslane to the body. Vitamin C is known to be vital for collagen while vitamin E plays a vital role in cell regeneration. These vitamins help to keep the skin free from blemishes.

Healthy Bone: Calcium, magnesium and phosphorus provided by purslane are essential minerals for strong and healthy bones. These minerals help to to prevent and treat osteoporosis and arthritis.

How To Use

Purslane's leaves, stems, and flower buds are very much edible and they are highly nutritious. Purslane can be used in salads and soups. It is good for stir-fries.

It is good to know that the fresh young leaves are the best for use.

Some people apply fresh purslane leaf on the skin to treat burns, and other skin ailments.

Side Effects

Enough data have not been recorded on the side effects associated with the use purslane.

NOTE

Amaranth Greens

Scientific Name: *Amaranthus dubious*

Overview

Amaranth Greens are herbaceous edible leafy vegetables that are native to Mexico and Central America. In the pre-Columbian time, it is one of the healthiest staple foods cultivated by the Aztecs and Incas.

Nowadays, it's mostly cultivated in the tropical climate of Asia, Latin America, and Africa where it flowers from some to fall.

In the subtropical environment, it can flower throughout the year.

In India, China, and Africa amaranth is usually cultivated as leafy-vegetable. The Europeans and Americans cultivate amaranth for their grains.

Health Benefits

- The stems and leaves contain a healthy amount of insoluble and soluble dietary fiber. This is why it is highly recommended by dieticians for a weight loss program and control of cholesterol levels in the body.

- Amaranth leaves are known to contain no zero cholesterol and a good amount of healthy fats. The greens contain approximately 23 calories/100g.

- Amaranth greens are vital for complete wellness of the body as they contain adequate amounts of antioxidants, vitamins, phytonutrients, and minerals required by the body.

- Iron is one of the essential components for the production of red blood cells. During cellular metabolism, iron serves as a co-factor for

cytochrome oxidase
(oxidation-reduction enzyme).
A fresh Amaranth green of
about 100g carries 29% DRI of
iron.

- Amaranth greens contain a
high amount of potassium,
even more than spinach.
Potassium is a very important
mineral in the cells and body
fluids. It helps to regulate
blood pressure and heart rate.

- It also contains high amounts
of magnesium, calcium,
manganese, zinc, and copper,
which are vital components for
the body cells.

- Like other greens, amaranth helps the body in preventing weakness of the bone, which is known as iron-deficiency anemia (osteoporosis).

How To Use
For the grain:

- Add to water twice the volume of the grain or 2.4 times the weight of the grain and boil.

For the leave:

- Separate the leaf and stem.

- Wash the leaf with cold water and gently pat dry with a tissue.

- Then chop before you use it in any recipe. It can also be used without chopping.

- Do not overcook the amaranth leaf so you don't destroy most of its nutrients, especially the vitamins and antioxidants.

- It can be used in soups, stews, curries, and mixed vegetable dishes.

- You can also use it raw to make juice or salad.

NOTE

CHAPTER 8

DR SEBI FOOD LIST

Vegetables

- ✓ Arame
- ✓ Wild Arugula
- ✓ Bell Pepper
- ✓ Zucchini
- ✓ Chayote
- ✓ Wakame
- ✓ Dulse
- ✓ Nopales
- ✓ Cucumber
- ✓ Garbanzo Beans
- ✓ Hijiki
- ✓ Sea Vegetables
- ✓ Avocado
- ✓ Dandelion Greens
- ✓ Izote flower and leaf
- ✓ Kale
- ✓ Cherry and Plum Tomato
- ✓ Mushrooms except Shitake

- ✓ Lettuce except iceberg
- ✓ Olives
- ✓ Nori
- ✓ Onions
- ✓ Purslane Verdolaga
- ✓ Squash
- ✓ Tomatillo
- ✓ Turnip Greens
- ✓ Amaranth
- ✓ Watercress
- ✓ Okra

Fruits

- ✓ Tamarind
- ✓ Prickly Pear
- ✓ Peaches
- ✓ Bananas
- ✓ Figs
- ✓ Prunes
- ✓ Cherries
- ✓ Berries
- ✓ Rasins
- ✓ Currants
- ✓ Pears
- ✓ Dates

- ✓ Orange
- ✓ Grapes
- ✓ Limes
- ✓ Mango
- ✓ Plums
- ✓ Apples
- ✓ Soft Jelly Coconuts
- ✓ Melons
- ✓ Cantaloupe
- ✓ Papayas
- ✓ Soursoups

Spices and Seasonings

- ✓ Sage
- ✓ Achiote
- ✓ Sweet Basil
- ✓ Basil
- ✓ Dill
- ✓ Habanero
- ✓ Cayenne
- ✓ Bay Leaf
- ✓ Onion Powder
- ✓ Oregano

- ✓ Pure Sea Salt
- ✓ Thyme
- ✓ Savory
- ✓ Cloves
- ✓ Tarragon
- ✓ Powdered Granulated Seaweed

- ✓ Rye
- ✓ Tef
- ✓ Amaranth
- ✓ Quinoa
- ✓ Wild Rice

Grains

- ✓ Fonio
- ✓ Spelt
- ✓ Kamut

Sugars and Sweeteners

- ✓ Sugar (gotten from dried dates)
- ✓ Agave Syrup gotten from

cactus
(100% Pur
e)

Herbal Teas

- ✓ Chamomile
- ✓ Red
  Raspberry
- ✓ Elderberry
- ✓ Fennel
- ✓ Burdock
- ✓ Ginger
- ✓ Tila

Nuts and Seeds

- ✓ Brazil Nuts
- ✓ Raw
  Sesame
  Seeds
- ✓ Hemp seeds
- ✓ Walnuts

Oils

- ✓ Avocado Oil
- ✓ Sesame Oil
- ✓ Coconut Oil

- ✓ Grapeseed Oil
- ✓ Hempseed Oil
- ✓ Olive Oil

OTHER BOOKS BY THE SAME AUTHOR

Dr. Sebi Mucus Cleanse

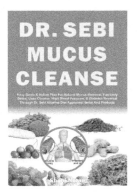

Link to kindle edition: https://www.amazon.com/dp/B08G4Z3D8H

Link to print edition: https://www.amazon.com/DR-SEBI-MUCUS-CLEANSE-Full-body/dp/B08GB253XW

Dr. Sebi Fasting For Weight Loss, Treatment And Cure

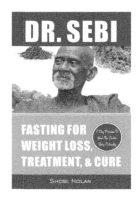

Link to kindle edition: https://www.amazon.com/dp/B08H1HXCSN

Link to print edition: https://www.amazon.com/SEBI-FASTING-WEIGHT-LOSS-TREATMENT/dp/B08GVGCDC2

Dr. Sebi Alkaline Diet Detox Guide For Women

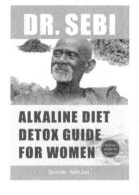

Link to kindle edition: https://www.amazon.co m/dp/B08H2FSSJ5

Link to print edition: https://www.amazon.co m/SEBI-ALKALINE-DETOX-GUIDE-WOMEN/dp/B08GVGD 18H

Dr. Sebi Natural Blood Pressure Control

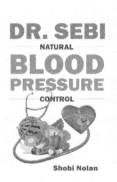

Link to kindle edition: https://www.amazon.co m/dp/B08JCKFNNL

Link to print edition: https://www.amazon.co m/SEBI-NATURAL-BLOOD-PRESSURE-CONTROL/dp/B08JB1X H13

Dr. Sebi Approved 3-Day Mucus Buster Diet For Women

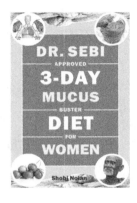

Link to kindle edition: https://www.amazon.co m/dp/B08GMBD8DX

Link to print edition: https://www.amazon.co m/APPROVED-3-DAY-MUCUS-BUSTER-WOMEN/dp/B08GVJTR NY

Dr Sebi 7-Day Cure For Herpes

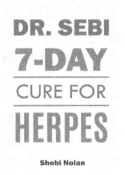

Link to kindle edition: https://www.amazon.co m/dp/B08KGYVP8M

Dr Sebi Easy Guide To Stop Drinking Alcohol

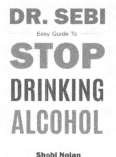

Link to kindle edition: https://www.amazon.co m/dp/B08KH2L5RZ

Dr Sebi Low Cholesterol Diet

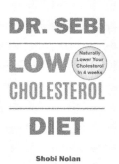

Link to kindle edition: https://www.amazon.co m/dp/B08KGZZKBP

Dr Sebi Easy Way To Stop Smoking

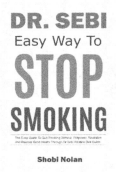

Link to kindle edition: https://www.amazon.co m/dp/B08J9QNZBR

Link to print edition: https://www.amazon.co m/SEBI-EASY-WAY-STOP-SMOKING/dp/B08JF5C ZBZ

Dr. Sebi Diet Guide To Stop Acid Reflux

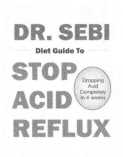

Link to kindle edition: https://www.amazon.co m/dp/B08JB29WD8

Link to print edition: https://www.amazon.co m/SEBI-DIET-GUIDE-STOP-REFLUX/dp/B08JF29R HF

The New Breath - Dr. Sebi's Natural Science To Stop Asthma

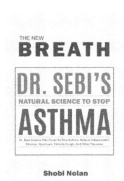

Shobi Nolan

Link to kindle edition: https://www.amazon.com/dp/B08JB565XR

Link to print edition: https://www.amazon.com/NEW-BREATH-Inflammation-Sinusitis-Heartburn/dp/B08JF5CS15

Dr. Sebi Alkaline Herbal Cure In 28 days

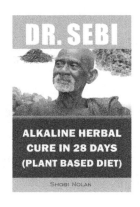

Link to kindle edition: https://www.amazon.com/dp/B08H1G3CQQ

Link to print edition: https://www.amazon.com/Sebi-Alkaline-Herbal-PLANT-BASED/dp/B08GVLWJVJ

The Dr. Sebi Diabetes Cure Book

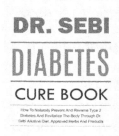

DR. SEBI

DIABETES

CURE BOOK

How To Naturally Prevent And Reverse Type 2
Diabetes And Revitalize The Body Through Dr.
Sebi Alkaline Diet, Approved Herbs And Products

Shobi Nolan

Made in the USA
Las Vegas, NV
23 November 2022